LAUGHTER THERAPY BENEFITS

A Complete Guide For Unveiling The Transformative Journey And Exploring The Profound Benefits From Giggles To Wellness

WALTER ZYAIRE

No part of this book may be reproduced, stored in a retrieval system, or transmitted in any form or by any means, electronic, mechanical, photocopying, recording, or otherwise, without the express written permission of the author, with the exception of small extracts in critical reviews or articles.

DISCLAIMER

The information in this book is intended only for general informational purposes; it should not be used in lieu of professional advice or medical care. Since the author is not licensed to practice therapy, the information offered should not be used in place of the expertise, judgment, or guidance of qualified mental health or medical professionals. Readers are encouraged to consult therapists, medical specialists, or other qualified authorities regarding their particular situation and needs. The publisher and author disclaim all liability for any actions or decisions taken by readers based on the information in this book. Results may vary from person to person and this book's approaches, procedures, and strategies may not be suitable in all circumstances. Considering unique situations and consulting a qualified expert are essential when choosing the right course of action. Neither the publisher nor the author recommend or guarantee the efficacy of any therapy or treatment that is indicated in this book. Because the information is based on the author's research and understanding at the time of publishing, it could not reflect the most recent developments or practices in the treatment area. The publisher and the author both disclaim all liability for the accuracy, completeness, or use of the material in this book. Readers bear full responsibility for the decisions and actions they choose in light of the information presented in this book.

TABLE OF CONTENTS

ABOUT THE BOOK

"Laughter Therapy Benefits" is a crucial manual that explores the various facets of laughing therapy and gives readers a thorough grasp of its importance in enhancing general well-being. The book delves into the historical foundations of laughter therapy, charting its development from traditional customs to contemporary acceptance. The book's goal and scope are established, which also stress the value of laughter for mental, physical, and emotional well-being.

The parts that follow explore the science of laughter and its health and psychological advantages. The substantial effects of laughter on pain relief, cardiovascular health, immune system strengthening, stress reduction, and cognitive well-being become clearer to readers. The examination of methods for laughter therapy, including clubs, yoga, and meditation, gives readers' useful skills for introducing humor into their everyday lives.

This book's focus on laughing therapy in a variety of contexts—such as workplaces, hospitals, and mental health settings—makes it stand out. Examining various cultural viewpoints on laughter, emphasis is placed on how laughter serves as a common social bond. The relationship between laughing and emotional health is also explored in the book, illuminating how laughter may be used as a coping strategy and an outlet for emotions.

The article gives readers useful advice on how to include laughing therapy in their daily routines so they can improve their well-being. The case studies and success stories that are included demonstrate the institutional and personal transformation that laughter therapy can bring about. The book also discusses the difficulties and disputes related to laughter therapy, including skepticism and moral dilemmas.

The book give readers a peek into prospective breakthroughs and developments in the field of laughing therapy by examining current and future research in this area. "Laughter Therapy Benefits" is an invaluable tool for anyone looking for a more all-encompassing approach to pleasure and health. It provides a plethora of information as well as helpful advice on how to use laughter's healing properties.

CHAPTER ONE

OVERVIEW OF LAUGHTER THERAPY BENEFITS

HISTORY AND SOURCES OF LAUGHTER THERAPY

Laughter therapy, sometimes referred to as laughter yoga or laughter meditation, is a therapeutic method that uses laughter's healing properties to enhance one's mental, emotional, and physical health. Laughter therapy has its origins in traditional Eastern medicine, where it was acknowledged as a powerful therapeutic aid. Throughout history, laughter has been connected to spirituality and overall well-being in ancient civilizations such as India.

But it wasn't until the 1990s that laughing therapy became formally recognized as an organized field of study, thanks in large part to the groundwork done by Indian physician Dr. Madan Kataria.

In 1995, Dr. Kataria created the Laughter Yoga movement by fusing deep breathing exercises with yoga. This novel method emphasized that the body cannot distinguish between purposeful and real laughter and sought to incorporate laughter into daily life, independent of outside stimuli. The movement gained traction fast and has since expanded throughout the world, with laughter clubs and therapeutic sessions being held in other nations. The development and cultural adaption of laughter therapy demonstrates its popularity and efficacy in promoting general well-being.

LAUGHTER IS ESSENTIAL TO WELL-BEING

The numerous benefits that laughter has for the health and psyche of a person are fundamental to its significance for overall well-being. Many people refer to laughter as a natural medication because it releases endorphins, which are the body's feel-good chemicals that can reduce stress and increase happiness right away.

Laughter also improves blood circulation and cardiovascular health by stimulating the cardiovascular system. Laughing works several muscle areas as well, making it a low-intensity workout that improves physical fitness.

From a psychological standpoint, laughing lowers cortisol levels and promotes relaxation, making it a potent stress reliever. In addition to fostering interpersonal interactions and a sense of community, it also promotes social ties and bonding. Laughter therapy recognizes the connection between mental and physical health and the substantial impact that a pleasant emotional state may have on general health. Laughing regularly is seen as a proactive strategy for mental toughness and stress reduction.

Furthermore, the tenets of mindfulness and mindfulness-based stress reduction (MBSR) are in line with laughter therapy. It invites people to embrace the present moment and laugh as a type of meditation that develops self-awareness and mindfulness. People can cultivate a more optimistic outlook, strengthen their emotional resilience, and generally live better lives by adding laughing to their everyday routines.

Laughing therapy has a long history based on antiquated customs and is now acknowledged as a useful instrument for fostering overall well-being. Its numerous advantages, which cover the mental, emotional, and physical aspects of health, make it significant. Laughter therapy is becoming more and more popular around the world, and this is because it helps to create a happier and healthier society.

CHAPTER TWO
COMPREHENDING LAUGHTER
THE STUDY OF LAUGHTER SCIENCE

Laughter is a fascinating and intricate human behavior that has strong biological and psychological roots. According to science, laughing is the result of a complex interaction between neurological and physiological factors. The limbic system of the brain, especially the amygdala, and hypothalamus, is essential for processing all emotions, including humorous ones. Neurotransmitters like dopamine and endorphins are released by the brain in response to something funny, which adds to the happy feelings that come with laughing.

Furthermore, laughing causes the body to go through several physiological changes. The distinctive sounds and facial expressions associated with laughing are produced by the rhythmic contractions of the facial muscles, the release of tension in the diaphragm, and the exhalation of breath. Laughter is a fascinating example of the mind-body connection, illustrating the complex ways in which our mental and physical states are interwoven. This is highlighted by the elaborate orchestration of neurological and physiological responses that occur during laughter.

LAUGHTER'S PSYCHOLOGICAL ASPECTS

Laughter has a variety of psychological purposes, which are reflected in its intricate involvement in human social and emotional experiences. Its social role as a universal language that cuts over linguistic and cultural divides is one important feature. A strong social bonding factor that strengthens ties between people is laughter. A pleasant social environment is facilitated by shared laughter, which strengthens social relationships and fosters a sense of camaraderie.

Moreover, laughing has a significant positive impact on mental health. It provides a brief respite and psychological comfort, acting as a coping technique in difficult circumstances. Laughing has been shown to have therapeutic benefits by lowering stress hormones, easing anxiety, and even elevating mood. Laughter therapy has become a well-established method in therapeutic settings for fostering mental health, with a focus on the role humor plays in building emotional resilience.

PHYSICAL ADVANTAGES OF LAUGHING

Laughing has several health benefits in addition to its psychological ones, which makes it an important component of overall well-being. Laughing works several different muscle groups, which eases stress and encourages relaxation. In addition to offering instant comfort, this bodily release helps regulate stress over the long term, which may reduce the likelihood of illnesses linked to stress.

There is a connection between laughter and cardiovascular health. Laughter mimics the heart rate increase and enhanced blood flow that accompanies aerobic exercise. This cardiovascular engagement highlights the connection between physical well-being and laughter and may eventually lead to improved heart health. Laughing also activates the respiratory system, improving lung function and supplying the body with oxygen.

Exploring the scientific, psychological, and physical aspects of laughing is necessary to comprehend it. This complex phenomenon emphasizes laughter as a comprehensive representation of the human experience with significant implications for mental and physical health, showcasing the complex interaction between mind and body.

CHAPTER THREE

THE PAST LAUGHTER THERAPY

TRADITIONAL METHODS

Laughter therapy has a long history that includes ancient practices, current development, and acceptance as a therapeutic strategy. It is also referred to as laughter yoga or laughter meditation. Several ancient societies understood the therapeutic value of laughter. For instance, the ancient Indian art of yoga is where the idea of using laughter as therapy originated. The interdependence of the mind, body, and spirit is emphasized in yogic philosophy, and laughter is considered a healthy, happy way to express oneself.

Similarly, the importance of laughter in fostering balance and health was recognized by traditional Chinese medicine. According to traditional Chinese medicine, emotions are vital for preserving physical health, and laughing was seen as a useful method for balancing the body's energy, or Qi.

The notion that laughter may be used as a comprehensive strategy for wellness was first established by these antiquated customs.

CONTEMPORARY GROWTH AND ACKNOWLEDGMENT

Thanks to Dr. Madan Kataria's groundbreaking work, laughter therapy has evolved and gained prominence in current times. Indian physician Dr. Kataria started the Laughter Yoga movement in the 1990s. Laughter yoga promotes happiness and relaxation by fusing deep breathing exercises with yoga poses. Dr. Kataria's method became well-known due to its beneficial effects on both mental and physical health.

Laughter therapy became more widely accepted in the medical community after several research demonstrated its possible advantages. According to scientific studies, laughing causes the body's endorphins, which are naturally occurring feel-good chemicals, to be released, which enhances well-being overall. Moreover, laughter has been connected to lowered stress levels, stronger immune systems, and better cardiovascular health.

IMPORTANT PEOPLE IN THE DEVELOPMENT OF LAUGHTER THERAPY

Another important person in the development of laughing therapy is American writer and journalist Norman Cousins, who popularized the notion that laughter may be therapeutic. In his book "Anatomy of an Illness as Perceived by the Patient," Cousins wrote about his own experience utilizing laughter to reduce pain. His work advanced knowledge of the mind-body connection and the potential therapeutic benefits of humor.

Laughter therapy spread to several wellness and medical environments as it gained popularity. Globally, leaders in certified laughter yoga emerged, leading laughter sessions in community centers, businesses, and classrooms.

Laughter therapy went beyond its original therapeutic goals to incorporate exercise and a means of fostering joy and social connection.

The development of laughing therapy from ancient customs based on philosophical and cultural ideas to the current understanding of its therapeutic potential is an intriguing journey. Prominent individuals such as Dr. Madan Kataria and Norman Cousins have been instrumental in influencing the development of laughing therapy and proving its beneficial effects on mental, emotional, and physical health. Laughter therapy is a living example of the long-held belief that laughing is a strong tool for enhancing overall health as well as a natural way to convey delight.

CHAPTER FOUR
METHODS OF LAUGHTER THERAPY
YOGA OF LAUGHTER

laughing therapy techniques are a broad category of methods intended to maximize the healing power of laughing for both mental and physical health. One well-known method is Laughter Yoga, an original and cutting-edge idea that blends deep breathing exercises with yoga poses. The goal of Laughter Yoga, which was created in the 1990s by Dr. Madan Kataria, is to intentionally laugh, no matter how one is feeling, to foster happiness and well-being. Based on the idea that the body cannot tell the difference between real laughter and fake laughter, this technique has similar positive physiological and psychological effects.

LAUGHING AS MEDITATION

Another method to harness the restorative power of laughing is to practice laughter meditation.

This technique involves people laughing mindfully, paying attention to the sound and feeling of laughter. Laughing is a common way for meditation practitioners to improve awareness, lower stress levels, and cultivate a happy outlook. To promote relaxation and emotional release, laughing meditation frequently entails guided sessions where participants are encouraged to explore different sorts of laughter, from planned to spontaneous.

COMEDY CLUBS

Laughter Clubs offer a safe and encouraging environment for people to get together and do laughing exercises. These clubs usually use a version of the Laughter Yoga paradigm, which includes breathing techniques, basic movements, and group laughter exercises. Laughter Clubs provide a nonjudgmental area for people to laugh together, fostering social interaction and emotional health. Frequent attendance at laughter clubs has been linked to better general health, lower stress levels, and happier moods.

INCLUDING LAUGHTER IN EVERYDAY LIVING

Embracing laughter as a wellness tool and valuing it as such are key components of incorporating laughter into daily life. This can involve adding humor to everyday activities, appreciating the small things in life, and actively looking for chances to laugh out loud. A more humorous everyday existence is achieved by strategies including taking laughter breaks throughout work hours, telling jokes to friends and family, and learning to face obstacles with humor. Including deliberate laughter in daily activities can improve mental and emotional health over time, fostering resilience and a more upbeat attitude in life.

Many different methods fall under the umbrella of "laughter therapy techniques," such as "laughter yoga," "laughter meditation," "laugh clubs," and purposefully incorporating laughter into everyday life.

These methods provide a variety of ways for people to benefit from the restorative properties of laughing, which promote social, emotional, and physical well-being. Laughter therapy is a holistic approach to health that can be used in a group or individual setting. It emphasizes the value of humor and joy in leading a balanced and meaningful life.

CHAPTER FIVE

THE HEALTH ADVANTAGES OF LAUGHING

REDUCTION OF STRESS

It has long been known that laughter is a potent stress reliever. Endorphins are feel-good hormones that our bodies release when we laugh and are natural stress relievers. Laughter also lowers stress hormone levels, such as cortisol and adrenaline. Laughing causes the body to relax, which enhances feelings of general well-being. Laughing can be a useful coping strategy in difficult circumstances, assisting people in reducing their stress levels.

IMMUNE SYSTEM BOOST

It's often known that laughing can enhance your immune system. Laughter strengthens the body's defenses against diseases and disorders by increasing the creation of immune cells and antibodies.

Regular laughter has been shown in scientific research to boost immune cell function and enhance the body's defenses against bacteria and viruses. Laughter plays a major role in immune system maintenance by lowering stress and fostering a happy mental state.

CARDIOVASCULAR HEALTH

The benefits of laughter extend beyond mental health to include improved cardiovascular health. Our blood flow increases when we laugh, which improves circulation. This increase in blood flow has the potential to improve blood vessel health and lower the risk of heart-related problems.

Laughter has been linked to lowered blood pressure and improved cardiovascular health overall, according to studies. Laughing is consequently a heart-healthy and enjoyable habit to get into regularly.

LAUGHING RELIEVES PAIN NATURALLY

Laughing has been shown to have pain-relieving effects. Laughing causes the brain to release endorphins, which have the dual benefits of improving mood and acting as natural painkillers. This might be especially helpful for people who are dealing with chronic pain disorders. Moreover, laughing releases stress and discomfort by relaxing the muscles. Including humor in a pain management plan can be an effective way to supplement conventional methods and improve the general quality of life for those who are experiencing different types of physical pain.

COGNITIVE ADVANTAGES

Laughing has advantages for the mind that go beyond the happiness it produces right away. Frequent laughter has been linked to enhanced mental clarity and cognitive performance. It increases the amount of oxygen that reaches the brain, which promotes mental clarity and creativity.

Moreover, laughing activates several brain regions and fosters neural connections, all of which are beneficial for preserving cognitive function as people age. Laughter's beneficial effects on stress levels and mood also contribute to a resilient and flexible mind, which is important in preventing or alleviating mental health problems.

It should be noted that laughing has numerous health advantages that affect both mental and physical health. Laughter turns out to be a simple yet powerful tool for creating a healthier and happier existence, whether it's by lowering stress, strengthening the immune system, encouraging cardiovascular health, easing pain, or improving cognitive performance. Including laughing in everyday activities can be seen as a proactive and pleasurable way to maintain overall health in addition to being a source of pleasure.

CHAPTER SIX

USING LAUGHTER THERAPY IN VARIOUS SITUATIONS

HEALTHCARE USING LAUGHTER THERAPY

Laughter therapy has become a popular complementary and alternative method in the field of healthcare for enhancing general well-being. The significant positive effects that laughter may have on one's bodily and emotional well-being are acknowledged in this therapeutic intervention. Laughter therapy is frequently used in healthcare settings as a component of a comprehensive patient care strategy.

Numerous physiological advantages of laughter have been demonstrated, including improved immunological function, improved cardiovascular health, and even decreased pain perception. Laughter therapy, in addition to its physiological benefits, tries to improve the mood in medical settings and build a sense of camaraderie between patients and healthcare professionals. Better patient outcomes and a more encouraging healing environment may result from this.

JOKING AROUND AT WORK

Laughter therapy in the workplace is an example of how employee well-being and its effects on morale and productivity are becoming increasingly important. Laughter therapy is becoming a more popular method used by organizations to reduce stress, foster team building, and improve overall job satisfaction. Joking around and having fun aren't the only ways that employees can laugh at work; some organized games and activities are meant to elicit real laughter.

This strategy can lessen stress at work, enhance team member communication, and foster a happier, more supportive workplace. Through cultivating a culture that prioritizes humor, companies want to improve worker satisfaction, lower turnover, and encourage a more positive work-life balance.

LAUGHTER TREATMENT FOR MENTAL ILLNESSES

The benefits of laughter therapy as an adjuvant treatment for mental health issues have come to light. The idea that laughter is a natural stress reliever and mood booster is the foundation for the therapeutic use of laughter in mental health settings. The body's feel-good chemicals, endorphins, are released when you laugh, and this might help you feel happier. Laughter therapy is frequently used in mental health treatment programs that target problems like anxiety, depression, and stress-related illnesses. Mental health specialists lead group laughter sessions that offer a safe, accepting environment for people to express themselves and find comfort in laughter. For those with mental health issues, the social component of laughter therapy can help fight feelings of isolation and build strong support networks.

It should be noted that laughing therapy crosses conventional borders and finds use in a variety of contexts, including mental health treatment, the workplace, and healthcare. Laughing is a valuable therapeutic technique that can enhance mental and physical health, strengthen social bonds, and build a more resilient and good society.

CHAPTER SEVEN

DIFFERENT CULTURAL VIEWS ON LAUGHING

CROSS-CULTURAL HUMOUR

A dynamic and diverse component of human communication, humor differs greatly between cultures. Understanding what is humorous or hilarious has its roots in cultural contexts and is shaped by past events, societal conventions, and values. Humor is an intriguing lens through which to examine cultural variation, as what is hilarious in one culture may not be in another. Language quirks, cultural allusions, and even how satire or irony is interpreted all add to the complex fabric of humor that exists around the world.

Different cultural perspectives on humor frequently show up in different ways, such as through spoken jokes, slapstick comedy, or even the enjoyment of wit. For example, societies with a high-context communication style might be more likely to use implicit or indirect humor, which calls for a thorough comprehension of common experiences and cultural clues. Low-context societies, on the other hand, could favor more overt humor that uses simple language and circumstances that are broadly accessible. Cultural differences in humor serve to both illustrate how context shapes comic expression and to show a range of tastes.

LAUGHING AS A MEANS OF SOCIALISATION

Laughter is potent social glue that cuts through language boundaries and cultural divides. A feeling of unity is formed when people find something funny together, strengthening social ties and dismantling obstacles.

Laughing can serve as a common language in social situations, fostering a sense of harmony and shared humanity. It acts as a nonverbal means of expressing happiness, acceptance, and a common appreciation of life's lighter moments.

Laughter is essential to maintaining social norms and group cohesiveness within cultural groups. Laughing together may be a symbol of acceptance and a means of fostering socialization and identity development. Jokes and humor that are specific to a group foster a sense of camaraderie among those who have a common understanding and appreciation of subtle humor. On the other hand, a mismatch in humor or a lack of shared laughing might draw attention to cultural differences or indicate a possible social separation.

Additionally, the cultural background affects which kinds of humor are acceptable in which social contexts. In certain cultural contexts, something that is deemed acceptable could be viewed as insulting or improper. Building strong connections and facilitating effective cross-cultural communication requires an understanding of the cultural nuances of humor.

Examining humor in various cultural contexts reveals a diverse range of humorous expressions shaped by sociological, historical, and linguistic variables.

Laughter is powerful social glue that helps people connect and create a sense of community. Understanding and valuing the many cultural viewpoints on laughter fosters more inclusive and peaceful interactions between other groups and improves cross-cultural understanding.

CHAPTER EIGHT

PLEASURE AND EMOTIONAL HEALTH

HAPPINESS AND LAUGHTER

Laughing is a key factor in affecting emotional health and a potent means of achieving happiness. Human physiology and psychology have a strong connection between happiness and laughter. Endorphins, or "feel-good" hormones, are released by our brains when we laugh and contribute to feelings of happiness and exhilaration. This physiological reaction strengthens the link between laughter and elevated emotions by generating a positive feedback loop. Moreover, laughing frequently creates social bonds with others, encouraging a sense of unity and shared delight, which raises happiness levels even higher.

LAUGHING AS A WAY TO LET GO OF EMOTIONS

Laughing is more than just entertainment; it's a powerful way to let go of feelings.

During stressful, tense, or depressing times, laughing serves as a cathartic release, giving pent-up feelings a way out. This phenomenon is closely related to the idea that people use humor as a coping mechanism to get through difficult emotional situations. Laughing can be therapeutic, assisting people in processing and letting go of bad feelings. Laughter serves as an organic and unplanned emotional release mechanism, promoting emotional stability and well-being.

LAUGHING YOUR WAY THROUGH DIFFICULTIES

The adaptive aspect of laughter as a human behavior is demonstrated by its function in helping people cope with adversity. Laughing is a coping strategy that crosses cultural and societal barriers as life's obstacles range from little stressors to major adversity. Laughter can offer a brief reprieve from the stress of difficult circumstances and a new outlook during trying times. It functions as a coping mechanism that encourages resilience and enables people to face challenges with a more positive attitude. Laughing together in public places can also strengthen ties among people and build a network of support that makes it easier to face and overcome obstacles.

There are several facets to the relationship between emotional health and laughter. Laughing not only makes people happier, but it also serves as a coping technique and a therapeutic outlet when faced with difficulties in life. Laughter has a dramatic effect on emotional health, which emphasizes its value as an easy-to-use, natural technique for building resilient and optimistic thinking.

CHAPTER NINE

USEFUL ADVICE FOR INCLUDING LAUGHTER THERAPY

LAUGHING ACTIVITIES

Laughter therapy, sometimes referred to as laughter yoga or laughter meditation, is a special and useful method for enhancing both mental and physical health. A key component of this therapeutic approach is including laughter exercises in your routine. The goal of these workouts is to make you laugh out loud, which has a lot of health advantages. In addition to increasing blood flow and enhancing blood vessel function, laughter also promotes the body's natural feel-good chemicals, endorphins, to be produced.

It is not necessary to have jokes or a particular kind of humor to participate in laughter exercises. It entails deliberate, voluntary laughing that is frequently sparked by diverse pursuits and lighthearted exchanges.

For example, participants can play games, clap in time to music, or take part in easy role-playing activities that make people laugh. The secret is to foster an environment where people can laugh without being forced to laugh at jokes or other outside stimuli.

ESTABLISHING A JOVIAL ENVIRONMENT

The success of laughing therapy sessions depends on the establishment of a laugh-friendly environment. This means creating an environment that encourages rest, optimism, and candid conversation. Think about adding whimsical touches to the space, including vibrant décor, cozy furniture, and even props that can give it a lively feel. Reducing formality makes people feel more comfortable and increases their readiness to participate in laughter exercises.

Creating a non-judgmental environment is also crucial to inspire others to laugh freely and let go of their inhibitions. People of various ages and backgrounds can benefit from laughter therapy since it is an inclusive approach. The effectiveness of laughing therapy sessions is largely attributed to the establishment of a welcoming and accepting environment.

INCLUDING HUMOUR IN EVERYDAY ACTIVITIES

The advantages of laughing therapy go beyond scheduled sessions when it is incorporated into everyday activities. Laughing moments can be incorporated into everyday life with a few easy activities. Incorporate humor into your everyday conversations, whether they take place in social situations, at business, or home. Tell jokes, anecdotes, or amusing stories to coworkers, friends, or family to foster moments of laughter.

Think about adding quick pauses for laughs to your routine as well. Whether you laugh with others or by yourself, dedicate a short period every day to deliberate laughing exercises. This could be watching a humorous video, playing games, or just laughing out loud without planning. These little bursts of laughing can be quite effective stress relievers, reducing tension and elevating mood.

Laughter therapy provides a comprehensive approach to overall health, including activities that involve laughing, setting up spaces that encourage laughter, and incorporating humor into everyday activities. People who adopt the concepts of laughter therapy might reap long-term advantages for their physical and mental well-being in addition to the immediate joy of laughing.

CHAPTER TEN

CASE STUDIES AND TRIUMPHANT NARRATIVES

PERSONAL NARRATIVES OF TRANSFORMATION

Narratives of transformation are frequently impactful pieces of writing that highlight the remarkable journeys of people conquering obstacles and becoming better versions of themselves. These stories demonstrate the fortitude, tenacity, and personal development that people might encounter in a variety of spheres of their lives.

Sarah's experience, who suffered from severe anxiety and depression for years, is one powerful example. Sarah started a journey of transformation with the help of self-reflection, therapy, and a caring community.

She discovered how to face her anxieties, question her self-defeating ideas, and progressively start again in her life. Sarah's tale highlights the value of asking for assistance and building a solid support network in addition to demonstrating the victory of the human spirit.

Another moving story is that of Mark, a career professional who felt unfulfilled and trapped in a boring routine. After realizing that something needed to change, Mark decided to follow his long-lost passion for photography. With persistence and commitment, he not only improved his abilities but also rediscovered his purpose in life. Mark's metamorphosis is evidence of the transforming potential of pursuing one's passions and accepting change.

These anecdotes highlight the role that self-awareness, resiliency, and goal-setting play in the process of transformation. They cultivate a mindset that views obstacles as chances for growth and change, inspiring others to have faith in their ability to adapt and improve.

LAUGHTER THERAPY'S SUCCESS IN INSTITUTIONS

Laughter therapy, sometimes referred to as laughter yoga or laughter meditation, has become a well-recognized and potent method for enhancing general well-being. Laughter therapy has been successfully incorporated into programs by a variety of institutions, from business organizations to healthcare facilities, and the results have been favorable in terms of both physical and mental health.

One noteworthy success story concerns a medical facility that offered laughing therapy to patients receiving treatment for long-term conditions as an adjunctive method. The addition of laughter sessions not only helped patients feel better emotionally but also made them more optimistic. The facility noticed that participants in laughter therapy reported significantly lower stress levels and improved general well-being.

Similar to this, a progressive business integrated laughing therapy into its employee health program in a corporate setting. Laughter sessions were a common activity that made the workplace more upbeat and united. Workers reported better interpersonal relationships, less stress, and higher job satisfaction. This result improved staff retention and productivity in addition to improving the culture of the workplace as a whole.

Laughter therapy was found to be a good motivator for change in many institutional success stories. Laughter may be used in institutional settings, demonstrating its versatility and ability to promote a more peaceful and well-being environment. These examples highlight the value of creative approaches to wellbeing across a range of institutions and demonstrate the beneficial knock-on effects that laughing therapy can have on people individually as well as in groups.

CHAPTER ELEVEN

OBSTACLES AND DEBATES IN LAUGHTER THERAPY

DISBELIEF AND REBUTTALS

Even while laughter therapy is widely used and accepted in some groups, it is nonetheless subject to criticism and skepticism. The scientific foundation of laughter therapy is one of the main areas of disagreement. Opponents contend that there is insufficient and frequently subjective empirical support for the therapeutic benefits of laughter. Though there is some evidence to support the positive physiological and psychological effects of laughter, the specific claims made by proponents of laughter therapy are frequently regarded as exaggerated or without sufficient evidence.

Furthermore, doubters cast doubt on the long-term effectiveness of laughter therapy and express questions about the uniformity of findings across various studies. Researchers and medical professionals debate the possibility of a placebo effect and the fleeting nature of benefits from laughter. Critics contend that to validate laughing therapy as a reliable and successful type of intervention, more thorough, controlled research is required.

Laughter therapy's commercialization is another area of doubt. Laughter therapy could be used for profit as it becomes more and more popular as a wellness trend. The commercialization of laughing therapy, according to some detractors, may oversimplify mental health problems and fail to sufficiently treat the underlying causes of psychological discomfort.

MORAL ASPECTS TO TAKE INTO ACCOUNT

Laughter therapy raises several ethical issues, including potential cultural insensitivity and the suitability of the therapeutic practice. The idea of "forced laughter" in certain laughter therapy sessions, when participants are urged to laugh even when they are not truly amused, raises ethical questions.

Critics contend that because people could feel under pressure to fit in with the group dynamics, which could cause them discomfort or anguish, this technique calls into question people's authenticity and consent.

Furthermore, there are significant cultural differences in the context of laughter, so what is viewed as therapeutic in one society may not be in another. Laughter therapy practitioners must be aware of cultural quirks and make sure their method is inclusive and polite. Ignorance of cultural differences can lead to inadvertent insensitivity or the reinforcement of prejudices.

Moreover, there are moral questions about the credentials of those who practice laughter therapy. With the increasing popularity of laughter therapy, there is a chance that unqualified people will start providing therapeutic services. The integrity of laughing therapy as a therapeutic modality depends on practitioners upholding ethical norms, having the necessary training, and placing a high priority on participants' well-being.

Doubts and moral issues surrounding laughter therapy emphasize the necessity of continued study, conscientious application, and sophisticated comprehension of cultural dynamics. By addressing these issues, laughter therapy can be used more ethically and credibly in a variety of contexts.

CHAPTER TWELVE

PROSPECTIVE DEVELOPMENTS

CURRENT RESEARCH IN LAUGHTER THERAPY

The many positive effects of laughter on mental, emotional, and physical health are still being investigated in the field of laughter therapy research. Researchers and medical professionals are exploring the neurological underpinnings of laughing to gain a better understanding of how it alters brain chemistry and relieves stress. Research on the long-term effects of laughter therapy for mental health issues like anxiety, depression, and even neurodegenerative diseases is growing.

Moreover, current studies are providing insight into the social dimensions of laughter therapy. Research is being conducted to determine whether laughter might improve interpersonal connections, fortify social ties, and foster a feeling of community. With a focus on enhancing general psychological well-being, researchers are investigating the function of laughing in group dynamics, professional settings, and community contexts as the area develops.

Research on the physiological consequences of laughter therapy is developing in addition to its psychological benefits. Research on how it affects the immune system, the cardiovascular system, and how pain is perceived is becoming more and more active. Gaining insight into how laughing affects certain physiological functions may lead to the creation of novel therapeutic approaches, including the application of laughter to treat a range of illnesses.

PROSPECTIVE NOVELTIES

The future of laughing therapy is being significantly shaped by technological breakthroughs, which are at the forefront of prospective innovations. Applications for augmented reality (AR) and virtual reality (VR) are being investigated as means of producing fully immersive laughing experiences.

With the help of these advances, people will be able to participate in therapeutic laughter exercises from the comfort of their own homes, increasing the accessibility of laughter therapy.

Furthermore, there is a growing body of research being done on the incorporation of artificial intelligence (AI) in laughing therapy. AI-powered chatbots and virtual friends that make people laugh and offer emotional support are in development. These developments have the potential to make laughing therapy more accessible to a wider range of people, particularly those who would have trouble obtaining conventional kinds of treatment.

Collaborations with different therapeutic modalities are another aspect of laughing therapy's developing field. Researchers are looking into integrative methods that incorporate yoga, mindfulness, and meditation with laughing therapy. These collaborative therapies target the mental, emotional, and physical facets of health to provide all-encompassing well-being solutions.

Laughter therapy is becoming more widely recognized and accepted in the medical community, and this is being shaped by continuing research as well as prospective developments that could make it a more individualized and easily available therapeutic tool for improving general well-being.